Healthy, Tasty Detox Juice Recipes Cookbook

Simple & Delicious Detox Juice Recipes for
a Healthy Body & Mind

BY

Stephanie Sharp

License Notes

Copyright 2019 by Stephanie Sharp All rights reserved.

No part of this Book may be transmitted or reproduced into any format for any means without the proper permission of the Author. This includes electronic or mechanical methods, photocopying or printing.

The Reader assumes all risk when following any of the guidelines or ideas written as they are purely suggestion and for informational purposes. The Author has taken every precaution to ensure accuracy of the work but bears no responsibility if damages occur due to a misinterpretation of suggestions.

WWWWWWWWWWWWWWWWWWWWWWWWWWWWWWWWWWWW

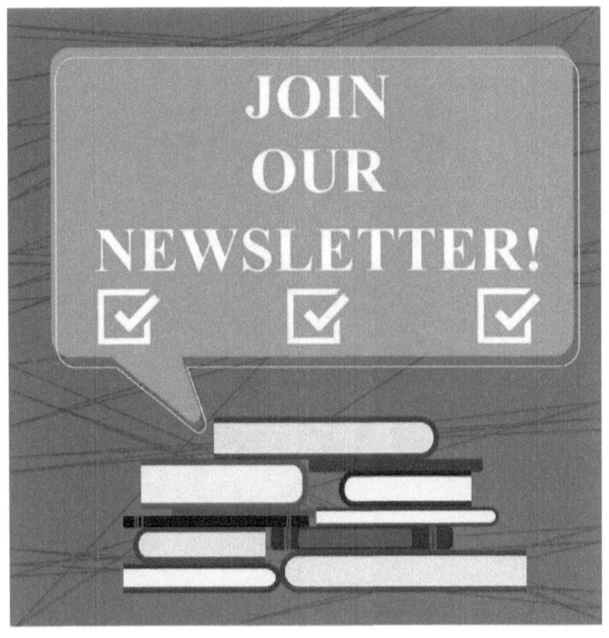

My deepest thanks for buying my book! Now that you have made this investment in time and money, you are now eligible for free e-books on a weekly basis! Once you subscribe by filling in the box below with your email address, you will start to receive free and discounted book offers for unique and informative books. There is nothing more to do! A reminder email will be sent to you a few days before the promotion expires so you will never have to worry about missing out on this amazing deal. Enter your email address below to get started. Thanks again for your purchase!

Just scan QR-code to get started!

wwwwwwwwwwwwwwwwwwwwwwwwwwwwwwwwwwwwwwwwwwww

Table of Contents

Introduction

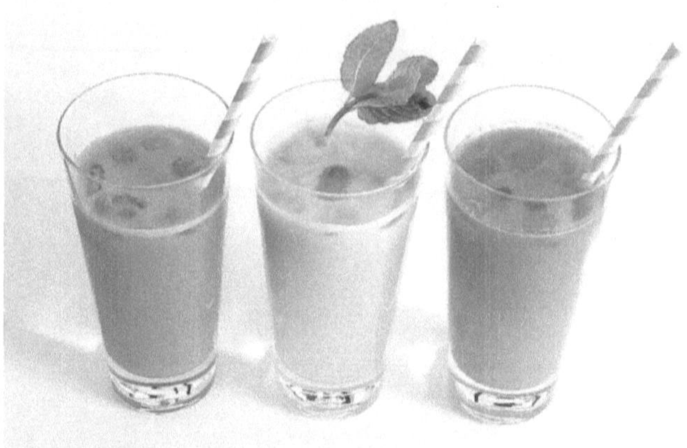

If you plan on detoxifying your body, the best way to do so is by juicing. When you ingest various types of junk food, you are packing your body with harmful chemicals that can affect your digestive functions on a day to day basis.

When delicious juices are made from home, you have the option to pack them with nutritious fruits and veggies of your choice which in turn fill your body with the required minerals and vitamins that your body requires to flush your system of bacteria and harmful chemicals.

You would be surprised to see the many benefits derived from an 8- ounce glass of homemade juice. You would not only lose some weight or gain energy; it goes far deeper than that.

As you peruse the 30 delicious recipes in this Healthy, Tasty, Detox Juice Recipes Cookbook you will discover how beneficial homemade juice really is for you as it soothes your mind and body.

Antioxidant Packed Orange Juice

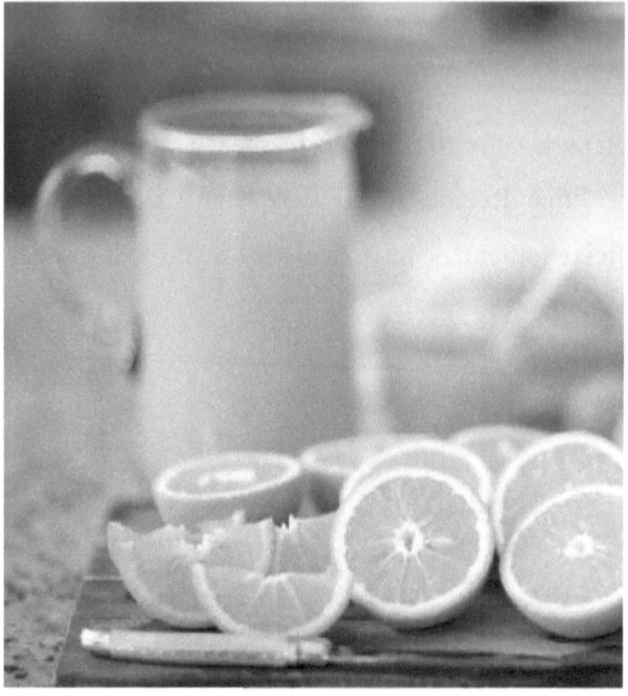

An all rounded Antioxidant Packed Orange Juice, sure to meet your requirements.

Serves: 1

Time: 5 mins.

Ingredients:

- Oranges (2, peeled)
- Carrots (3, fresh, peeled)
- Cucumbers (2, fresh, seedless)
- Bell Pepper (1, yellow, deseeded)
- Ginger (1 piece, fresh and peeled)

Directions:

1. Thoroughly wash ingredients under running water and use hands to scrub.

2. In a juicer add freshly washed ingredients and begin to juice.

3. Pour mixture into a suitable sized glass and serve immediately.

Ultimate Cabbage Stomach Soother

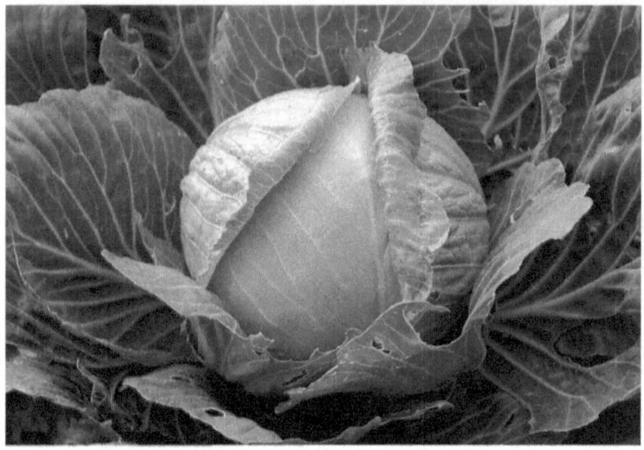

This Cabbage stomach soother is the ultimate concoction.

Serves: 1

Time: 5 mins.

Ingredients:

- Cabbage (¼ head, fresh, green)
- Kale (4 leaves, Fresh, torn)
- Celery (2 stalks, fresh)
- Apples (2, green, small)
- Ginger (½ of a slice, Fresh, peeled)

Directions:

1. Thoroughly wash ingredients under running water and use hands to scrub.

2. In a juicer add ingredients and blend.

3. Pour mixture into a suitable sized glass (chilled) and serve immediately.

Green Power Juice

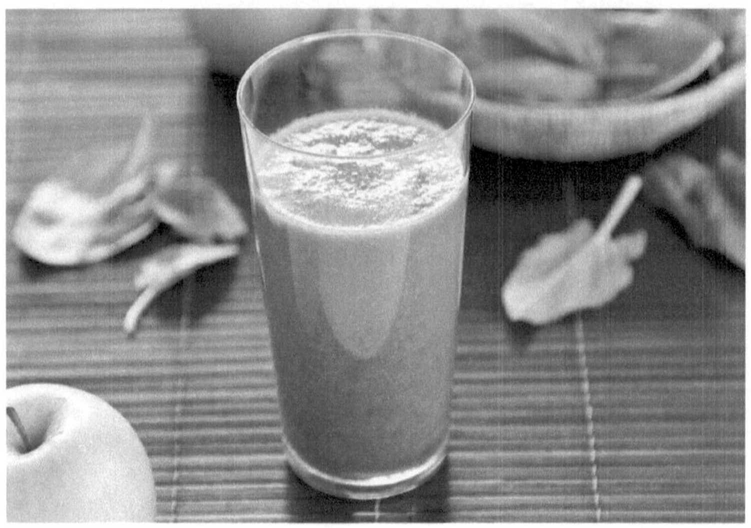

This concoction is not just delicious but is packed with iron and antioxidants.

Serves: 1

Time: 5 mins.

Ingredients:

- Mint Leaves (1 bunch, small, fresh)
- Lime (1, fresh, peeled)
- Apple (1, fresh, green, cored)
- Cucumber (1, fresh and seedless)
- Cabbage (¼ head, fresh, green, torn)

Directions:

1. Thoroughly wash ingredients under water and use hands to scrub.

2. In a juicer add freshly washed ingredients and begin to juice.

3. Pour mixture into a tall glass, chill and serve immediately.

Wheatgrass Kiwi

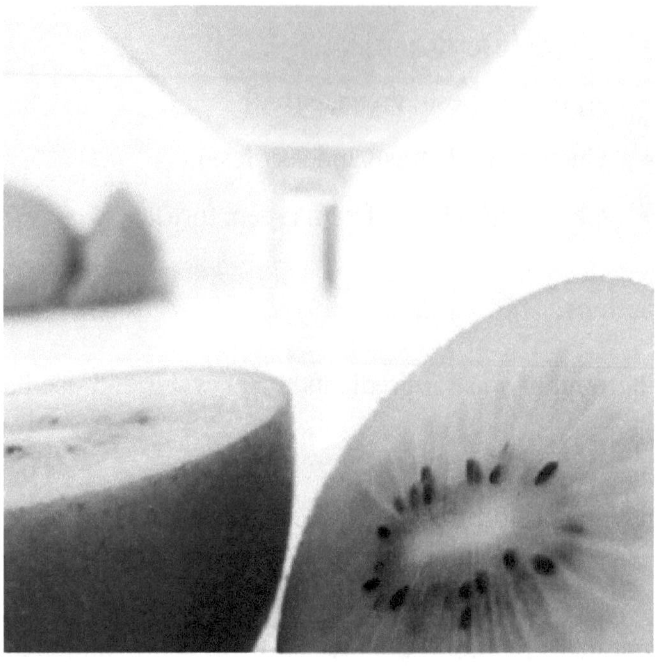

This wheatgrass Kiwi is a natural cleanser and will help you to start your day fresh and healthy.

Serves: 2

Time: 15 mins.

Ingredients:

- Rhubarb (2 stalks)
- Wheatgrass (½ handful)
- Kiwis (4)
- Cabbage (1 head)
- Lettuce (1 head)
- Bell pepper (½, green or red)
- Nectarine (1)
- Cherries (1 cup)
- Dandelion root (1)
- Dates (2)

Directions:

1. Thoroughly wash ingredients under water and use hands to scrub.

2. In a juicer add freshly washed ingredients and begin to juice.

3. Pour mixture into a tall glass, chill and serve immediately.

Peach and Fresh Ginger

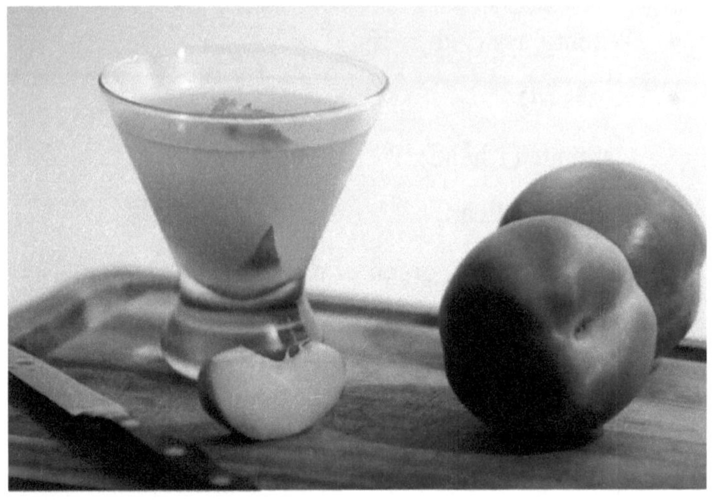

This Peach and Fresh Ginger detox juice combines fresh ginger with fresh peach making it the ultimate concoction.

Serves: 2

Time: 8 mins.

Ingredients:

- Strawberries (1 cup)
- Peaches (2)
- Ginger (½ slice, fresh)
- Broccoli (½ cup)
- Dandelion root (1)
- Mango (½)
- Potatoes (2, sweet)
- Papaya (1)
- Pomegranate (1)
- Cauliflower (1 head)

Directions:

1. Thoroughly wash ingredients under water and use hands to scrub.

2. In a juicer add freshly washed ingredients and begin to juice.

3. Pour mixture into a tall glass, chill and serve immediately.

Four Seasons Detox Juice

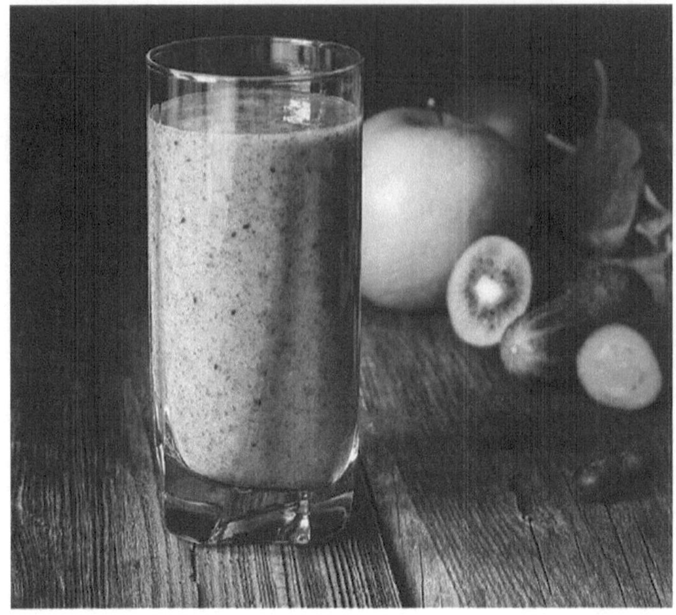

Naturally sweet Detox Juice recipe packed with apples, ginger and vegetables, fit for all seasons.

Serves: 1

Time: 4 mins.

Ingredients:

- Apple (1, fresh, red)
- Cabbage (½ head, fresh, torn)
- Pepper (green, seeded)
- Parsley (3 sprigs, fresh)
- Broccoli (4-5 florets, fresh, washed)
- Ginger (1 piece, fresh, peeled)

Directions:

1. Thoroughly wash ingredients under water and use hands to scrub.

2. In a juicer add freshly washed ingredients and begin to juice.

3. Pour mixture into a tall glass, chill and serve immediately.

Tasty Tomatillo Juice

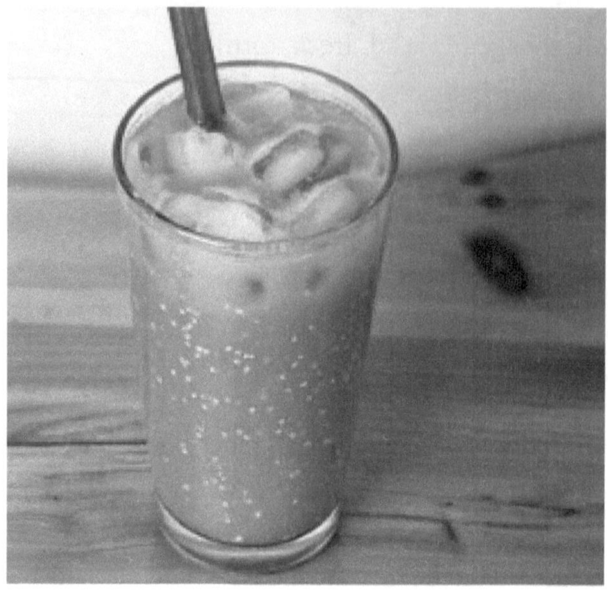

A refreshing concoction that is not just healthy but delicious.

Serves: 1 Glass

Time: 4 mins.

Ingredients:

- Tomatillos (3, fresh, skin removed)
- Carrots (5, fresh and peeled)
- Apple (1, green, cored)
- Basil (1 sprig, green, fresh)
- Ginger (1 piece, fresh, peeled)

Directions:

1. Thoroughly wash ingredients under water and use hands to scrub.

2. In a juicer add freshly washed ingredients and begin to juice.

3. Pour mixture into a tall glass, chill and serve immediately.

Easy Sun Juice

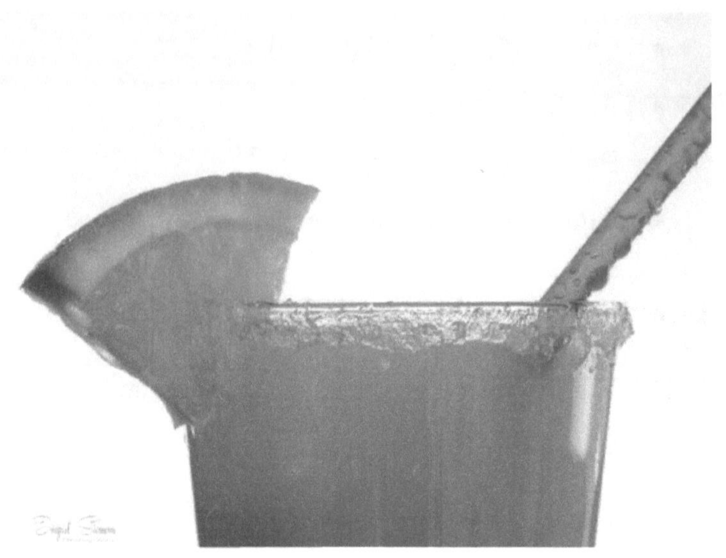

A powerful detox juice consisting of turmeric, lemon, orange, beet, ginger when combined creates a strong antioxidant.

Serves: 1

Time: 4 mins.

Ingredients:

- Orange (1, fresh and peeled)
- Lemon (1, fresh and peeled)
- Carrot (1, fresh and purple)
- Carrot (1, large, peeled)
- Beet (1, Fresh, Peeled)
- Ginger (1 piece, fresh and peeled)
- Turmeric (1 piece, fresh and peeled)

Directions:

1. Thoroughly wash ingredients under water and use hands to scrub.

2. In a juicer add freshly washed ingredients and begin to juice.

3. Pour mixture into a tall glass, chill and serve immediately.

Easy Radish and Pear Juice

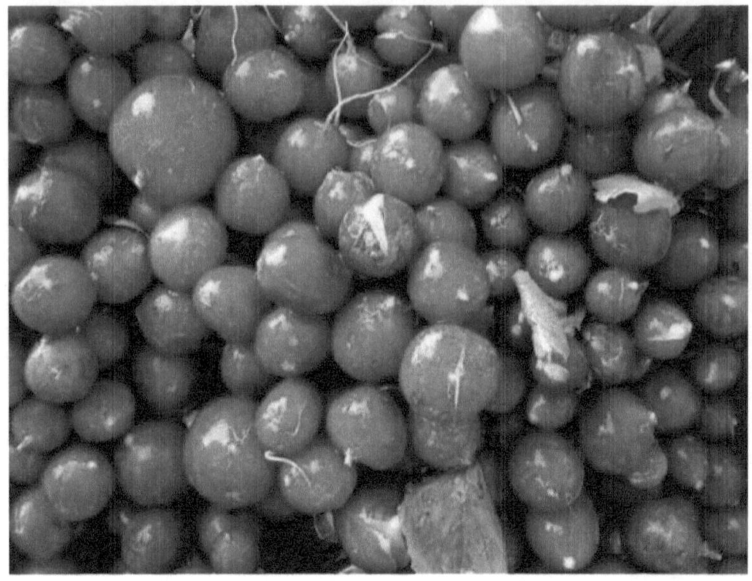

A delicious and healthy detoxifying recipe that is sure to get the job done.

Serves: 2

Time: 7 mins.

Ingredients:

- Arugula (1 bunch, fresh, torn)
- Radishes (3, green parts removed)
- Carrots (3, fresh, peeled)
- Celery (3, fresh, stalks)
- Cucumber (1/3, fresh, seedless)
- Pear (1, fresh, cored)
- Ginger (1 piece, fresh, peeled)

Directions:

1. Thoroughly wash ingredients under water and use hands to scrub.

2. In a juicer add freshly washed ingredients and begin to juice.

3. Pour mixture into a tall glass, chill and serve immediately.

Summertime Mint and Papaya Cooler

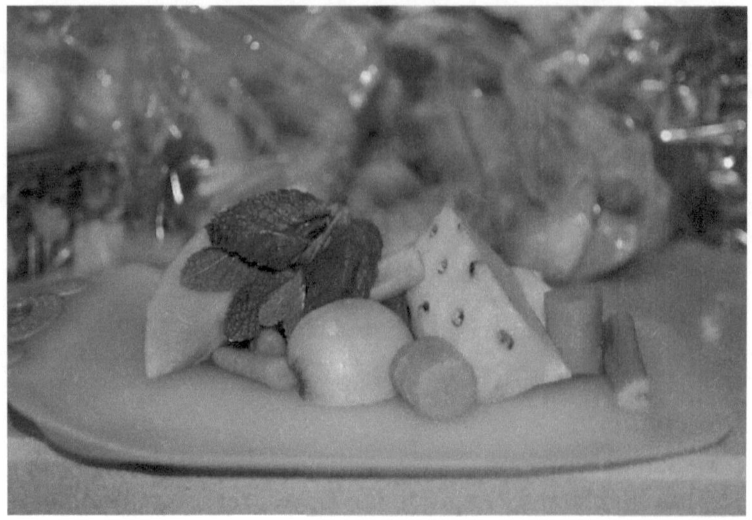

A healthy detox juice recipe that combines summertime mint with papaya which is not just refreshing but is a great antioxidant.

Serves: 2

Time: 5 mins.

Ingredients:

- Papaya (¼, peeled, deseeded)
- Apples (2, fresh, cored)
- Cucumber (1, fresh, large, seedless)
- Mint (1 bunch, fresh, torn)

Directions:

1. Thoroughly wash ingredients under water and use hands to scrub.

2. In a juicer add freshly washed ingredients and begin to juice.

3. Pour mixture into a tall glass, chill and serve immediately.

Chard Style Café Juice

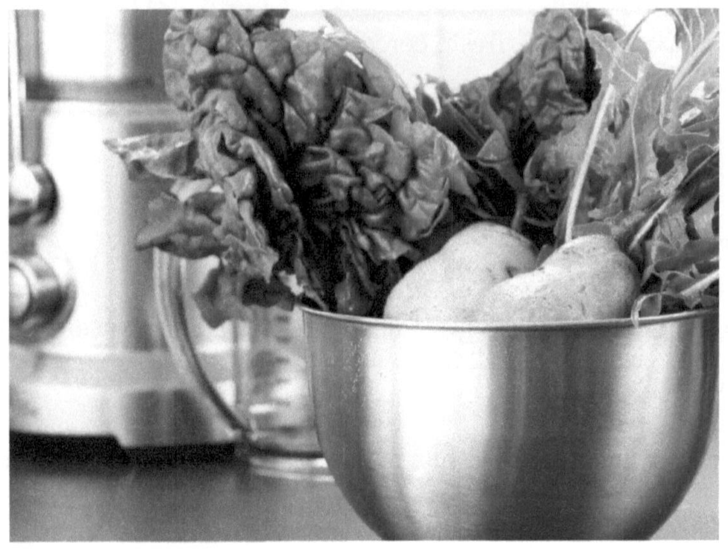

A beneficial and refreshing recipe that is sure to give the body a good detox.

Serves: 1

Time: 5 mins.

Ingredients:

- Carrots (3, fresh, peeled)
- Cucumber (1, fresh, seedless)
- Lemon (½, fresh, peeled)
- Chard (2, leaves, large, torn)
- Oregano (2 sprigs, stems, Leaves removed)

Directions:

1. Thoroughly wash ingredients under water and use hands to scrub.

2. In a juicer add freshly washed ingredients and begin to juice.

3. Pour mixture into a tall glass, chill and serve immediately.

Green Pineapple Juice

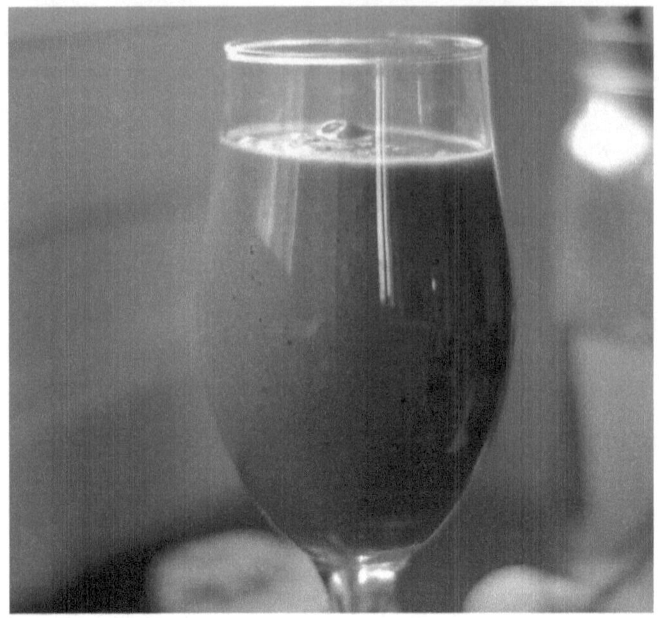

A healthy and delicious recipe that combines pineapple with kale, celery and basil leaves.

Serves: 2

Time: 4 mins.

Ingredients:

- Grapefruit (½, fresh, peeled)
- Lime (1, fresh, peeled)
- Pineapple (¼, Fresh)
- Kale (6 leaves, large, torn)
- Celery (2 stalks, Fresh)
- Basil Leaves (1 bunch, fresh, torn)

Directions:

1. Thoroughly wash ingredients under water and use hands to scrub.

2. In a juicer add freshly washed ingredients and begin to juice.

3. Pour mixture into a tall glass, chill and serve immediately.

Summertime Parsley and Squash Juice

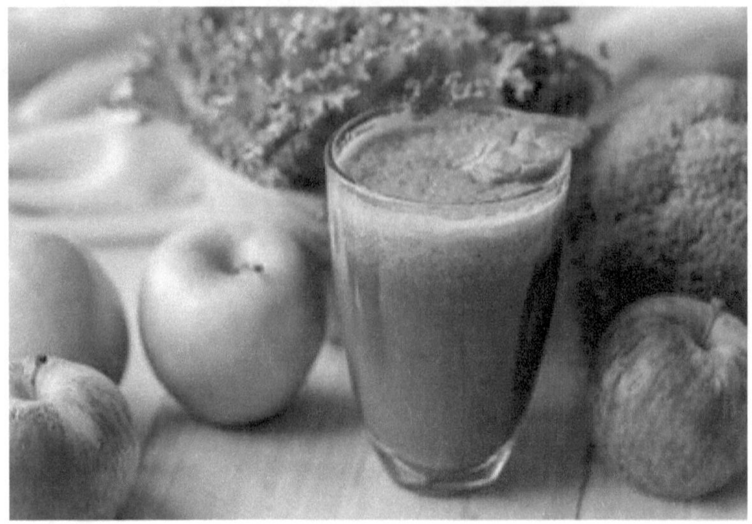

A naturally sweetened detox recipe that is sure to work miracles.

Serves: 1

Time: 5 mins.

Ingredients:

- Cucumber (½, fresh and seedless)
- Squash (1, fresh)
- Fennel Bulb (½)
- Apple (1, large, fresh, cored)
- Parsley (4 sprigs, fresh and torn)
- Ginger (1 piece, fresh and peeled)
- Lemon (½, Peeled)

Directions:

1. Thoroughly wash ingredients under water and use hands to scrub.

2. In a juicer add freshly washed ingredients and begin to juice.

3. Pour mixture into a tall glass, chill and serve immediately.

Classic Sweet and Sour Juice

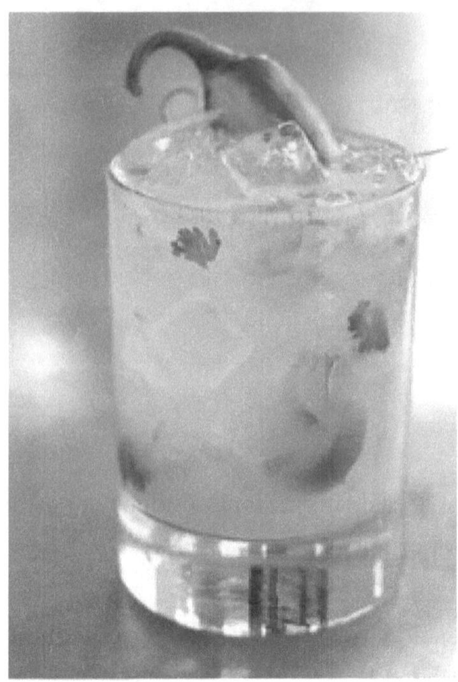

This Classic Sweet and Sour juice recipe is an all-time classic it is known for its miraculous detoxifying properties.

Serves: 2

Time: 4 mins.

Ingredients:

- Oranges (2, fresh, peeled)
- Grapefruit (1, fresh, peeled)
- Lemons (2, Fresh, peeled)
- Turmeric (1 piece, peeled)

Directions:

1. Thoroughly wash ingredients under water and use hands to scrub.

2. In a juicer add freshly washed ingredients and begin to juice.

3. Pour mixture into a tall glass, chill and serve immediately.

Antioxidant Packed Juice

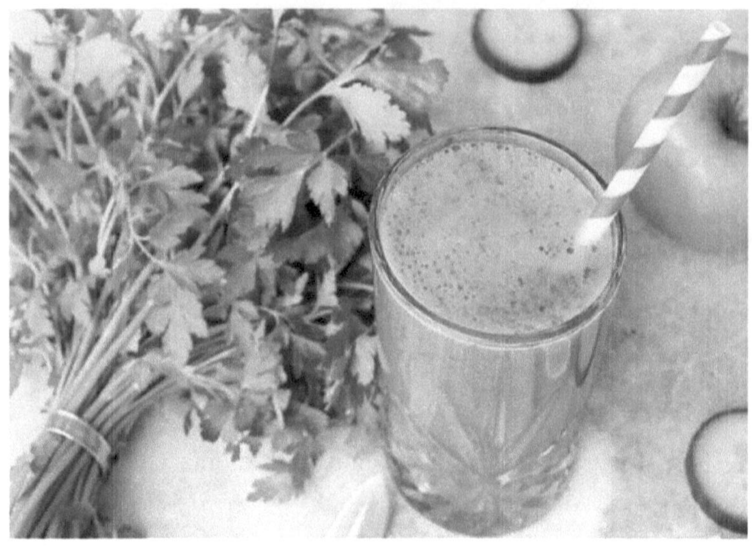

This recipe is packed with various detoxifying ingredients and the combination forms a great cleanser.

Serves: 2

Time: 3 mins.

Ingredients:

- Cabbage (¼ head, fresh, red)
- Rosemary (1 sprig, fresh, torn)
- Ginger (½ slice, fresh, peeled)
- Oranges (2, fresh, peeled)
- Beet (1, fresh)

Directions:

1. Thoroughly wash ingredients under water and use hands to scrub.

2. In a juicer add freshly washed ingredients and begin to juice.

3. Pour mixture into a tall glass, chill and serve immediately.

Spicy Carrot and Apple Juice

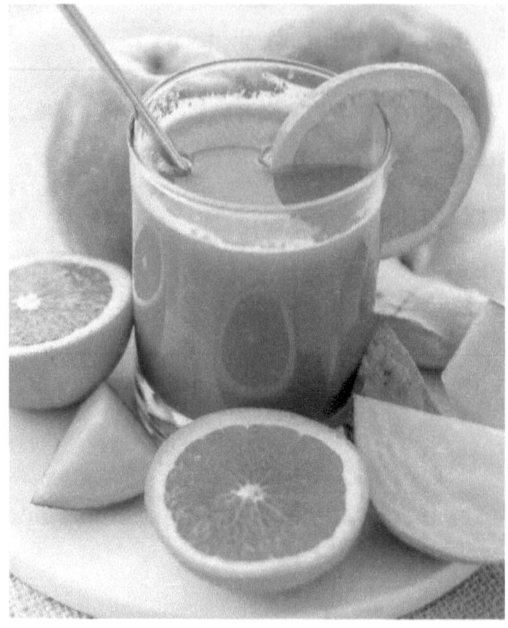

This Spicy Carrot and Apple Juice recipe is rich and healthy. The carrots and apples complement each other well.

Serves: 1

Time: 5 mins.

Ingredients:

- Carrots (3, fresh, large)
- Apples (2, fresh)
- Celery (2 stalks. Fresh)
- Ginger (1 piece, fresh, peeled)
- Turmeric (¼ inch, fresh, peeled)
- Cinnamon (dash, ground)
- Nutmeg (dash, round)

Directions:

1. Thoroughly wash ingredients under water and use hands to scrub.

2. In a juicer add freshly washed ingredients and begin to juice.

3. Pour mixture into a tall glass, chill and serve immediately.

Spicy Red Pepper Juice

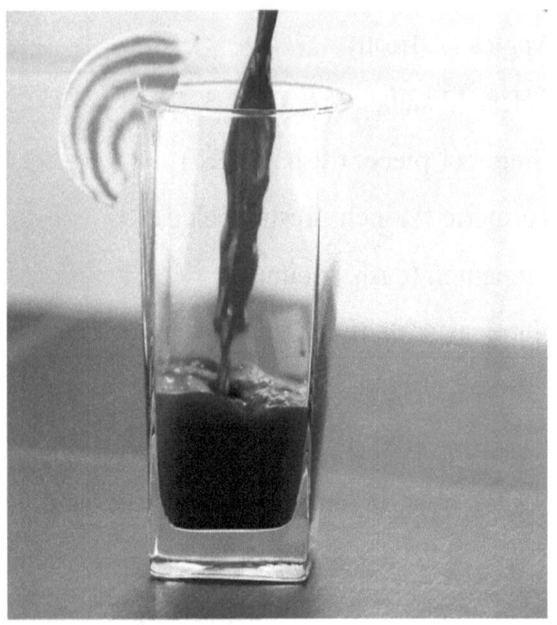

A spicy recipe that consist of bell peppers, cucumber, broccoli etc. It has a bunch of heat but is spicy and refreshing.

Serves: 2

Time: 10 mins.

Ingredients:

- Bell Peppers (2, red, chopped)
- Cucumbers (fresh and finely diced0
- Broccoli (2 bunches, fresh, torn)
- Carrots (2, peeled, diced)
- Jicama (1 cup, peeled, diced)
- Lime (1 cup, fresh)
- Basil (2 handfuls, fresh, torn)
- Tabasco Sauce (1-4 drops)
- Chia seed (2 tbsp)

Directions:

1. Thoroughly wash ingredients under water and use hands to scrub.

2. In a juicer add freshly washed ingredients and begin to juice.

3. Pour mixture into a tall glass, chill and serve immediately.

Calcium Packed Cucumber Juice

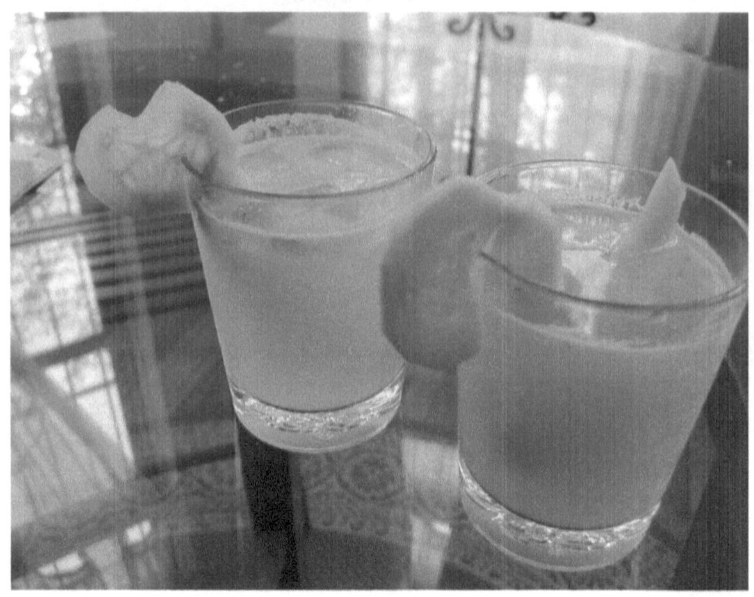

A nutritious recipe consisting of pineapple, celery, cucumber and lime, this juice is packed with calcium.

Serves: 1

Time: 4 mins.

Ingredients:

- Pineapple (¼, fresh, peeled)
- Celery (4 stalks, fresh)
- Cucumber (1, large, fresh and Seeds removed)
- Lime (1, fresh, peeled)

Directions:

1. Thoroughly wash ingredients under water and use hands to scrub.

2. In a juicer add freshly washed ingredients and begin to juice.

3. Pour mixture into a tall glass, chill and serve immediately.

Fruity Tonic Juice

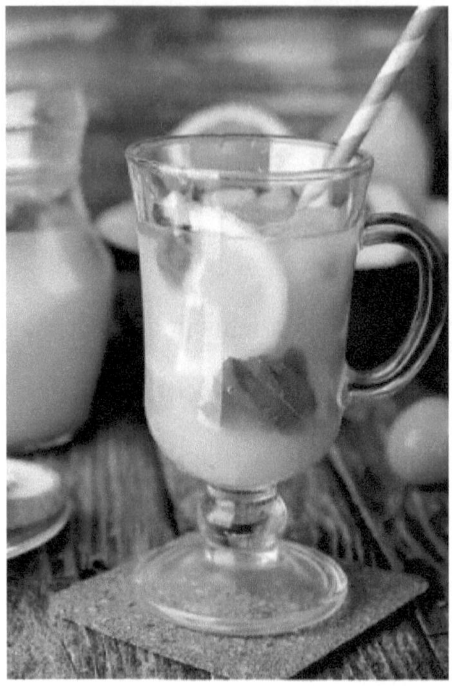

The fruits in this tonic juice is what gives it its unique color, this tonic juice is filled with vitamin c and bioflavonoids.

Serves: 1

Time: 5 mins.

Ingredients:

- Cantaloupe (¼, fresh, rind removed)
- Grapefruit (1, fresh, peeled)
- Lemon (1, fresh, peeled)
- Ginger (½ piece, peeled, diced)
- Turmeric (½ piece, peeled, diced)

Directions:

1. Thoroughly wash ingredients under water and use hands to scrub.

2. In a juicer add freshly washed ingredients and begin to juice.

3. Pour mixture into a tall glass, chill and serve immediately.

Bright Colored Purple Kale Juice

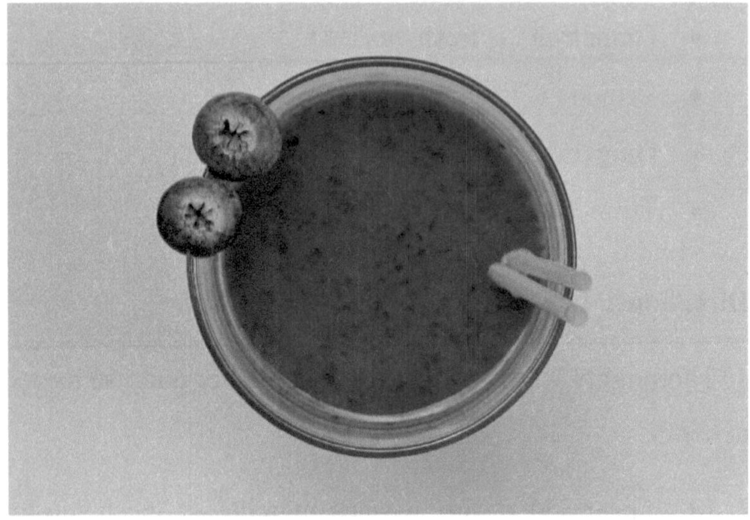

This nutritious recipe is a vitamin packed concoction that has great detoxifying properties.

Serves: 1

Time: 4 mins.

Ingredients:

- Kale (4 leaves, purple, torn)
- Carrots (6, large, peeled)
- Clementines (2, peeled)
- Lemon (fresh, peeled)
- Ginger (1 piece, fresh, peeled)

Directions:

1. Thoroughly wash ingredients under water and use hands to scrub.

2. In a juicer add freshly washed ingredients and begin to juice.

3. Pour mixture into a tall glass, chill and serve immediately.

Eggplant Watermelon

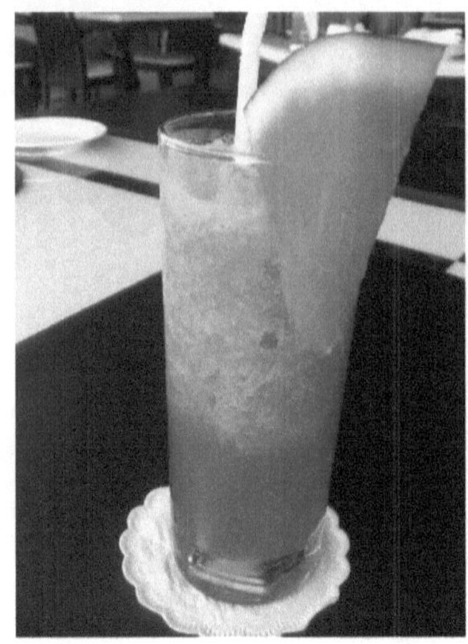

A healthy recipe that combines watermelon with eggplant creating an incredible detox juice.

Serves: 2

Time: 12 mins.

Ingredients:

- Cantaloupe (½)
- Eggplant (½)
- Watermelon (1 ½ cup)
- Peaches (2)
- Tomatoes (2)
- Potatoes (2, sweet)
- Carrots (4)
- Asparagus spears (2)
- Bell pepper (1 green, red)
- Rhubarb (1 stalk)

Directions:

1. Thoroughly wash ingredients under water and use hands to scrub.

2. In a juicer add freshly washed ingredients and begin to juice.

3. Pour mixture into a tall glass, chill and serve immediately.

Green Protein Juice

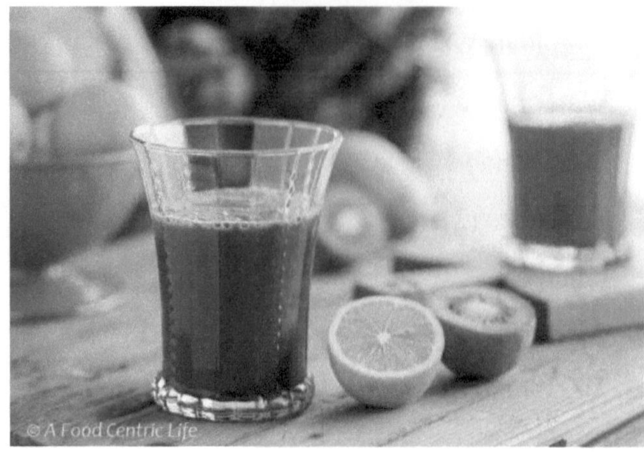

A magnificent green juice recipe that utilizes protein filled ingredients which the body needs for a good detox.

Serves: 1

Time: 5 mins.

Ingredients:

- Torn (4 leaves, fresh, torn)
- Swiss Chard (4 leaves, fresh, torn)
- Celery (4 stalks, fresh)
- Spinach Leaves (1 bunch, large)
- Lime (1, fresh, peeled)
- Apples (2, green, cored)
- Ginger (1 piece, fresh, peeled)

Directions:

1. Thoroughly wash ingredients under water and use hands to scrub.

2. In a juicer add freshly washed ingredients and begin to juice.

3. Pour mixture into a tall glass chilled and serve immediately.

Spiced Tomato Juice

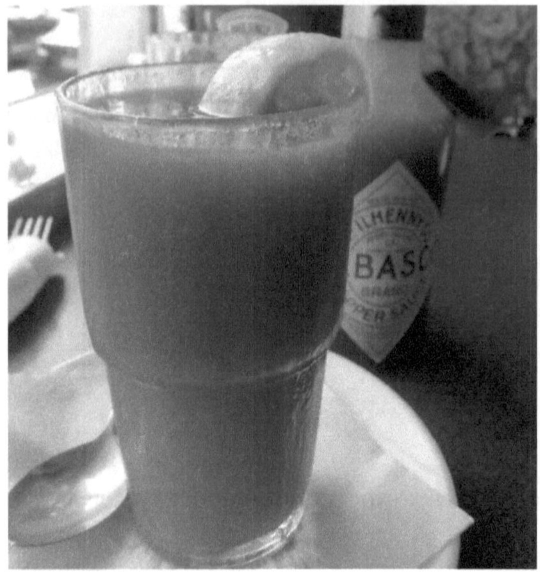

This spiced tomato juice recipe is a refreshing drink filled with antioxidants, enzymes and loaded with nutrients.

Serves: 2

Time: 7 mins.

Ingredients:

- Tomatoes (3, large, fresh)
- Celery (3 stalks, fresh)
- Carrots (2, large, fresh, peeled)
- Chiles (2, fresh)

Directions:

1. Thoroughly wash ingredients under water and use hands to scrub.

2. In a juicer add freshly washed ingredients and begin to juice.

3. Pour mixture into a tall glass chilled and serve immediately.

Golden Beat Juice

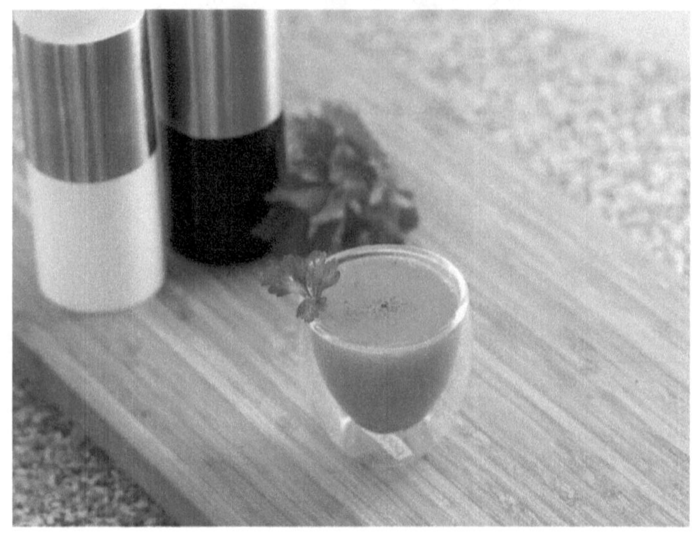

Beetroots are healthy, versatile vegetables that play a vital role in the detoxifying process.

Serves: 1

Time: 5 mins.

Ingredients:

- Beets (2, gold, peeled)
- Golden Beet (Leaves)
- Pineapple (¼, peeled)
- Lemon (1, fresh, peeled)
- Ginger (½, fresh, peeled)

Directions:

1. Thoroughly wash ingredients under water and use hands to scrub.

2. In a juicer add freshly washed ingredients and begin to juice.

3. Pour mixture into a tall glass, chill and serve immediately.

Tomato Madness Juice

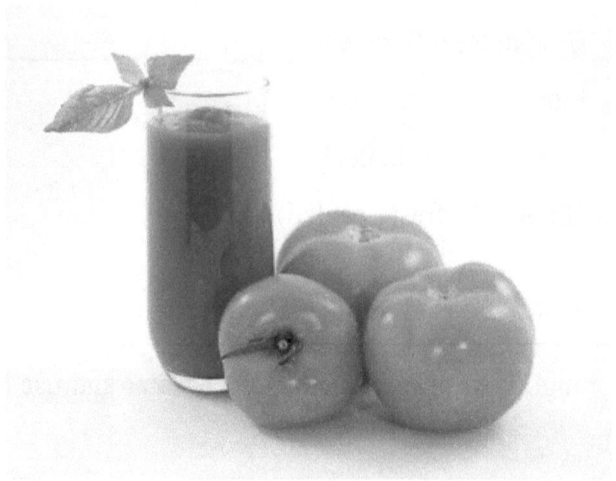

A nutrient filled, refreshing recipe that utilizes tomatoes, orange, carrots etc.

Serves: 1

Time: 5 mins.

Ingredients:

- Orange (1, fresh, peeled)
- Carrots (2, fresh, large, peeled)
- Bell Pepper (1, orange, destemmed, deseeded)
- Celery (2 stalks, fresh)
- Cucumber (½, fresh)
- Tomatoes (2, medium, chopped)

Directions:

1. Thoroughly wash ingredients under water and use hands to scrub.

2. In a juicer add freshly washed ingredients and begin to juice.

3. Pour mixture into a tall glass, chill and serve immediately.

Mediterranean Style Thyroid Juice

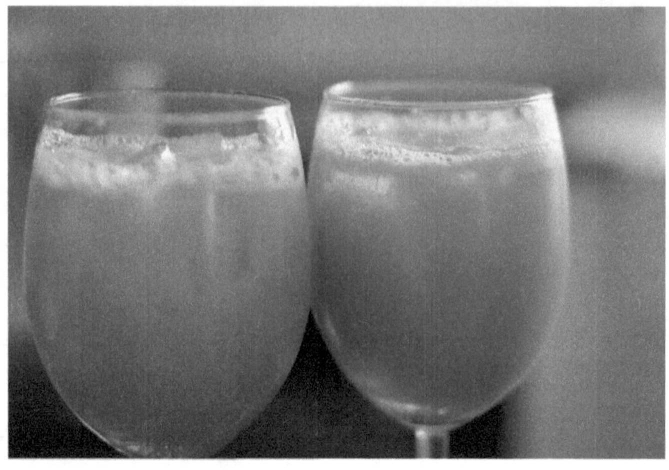

If you are seeking a gentle detox, this Mediterranean style Thyroid Juice recipe is the right one.

Serves: 1

Time: 4 mins.

Ingredients:

- Pepper (1, red, deseeded and destemmed)
- Tomato (1, fresh)
- Lemon (1, fresh, peeled)
- Cucumber (1, peeled)
- Oregano (4 leaves, fresh, roughly)
- Sea Salt (dash)

Directions:

1. Thoroughly wash ingredients under water and use hands to scrub.

2. In a juicer add freshly washed ingredients and begin to juice except for the oregano leaves, dash of sea salt and a slice of lemon.

3. For the tastiest experience it is recommended that you wrap your oregano around your cucumber for burst of flavor.

4. Pour mixture into two tall glasses, chill and serve immediately.

Simple Mint and Peach Juice

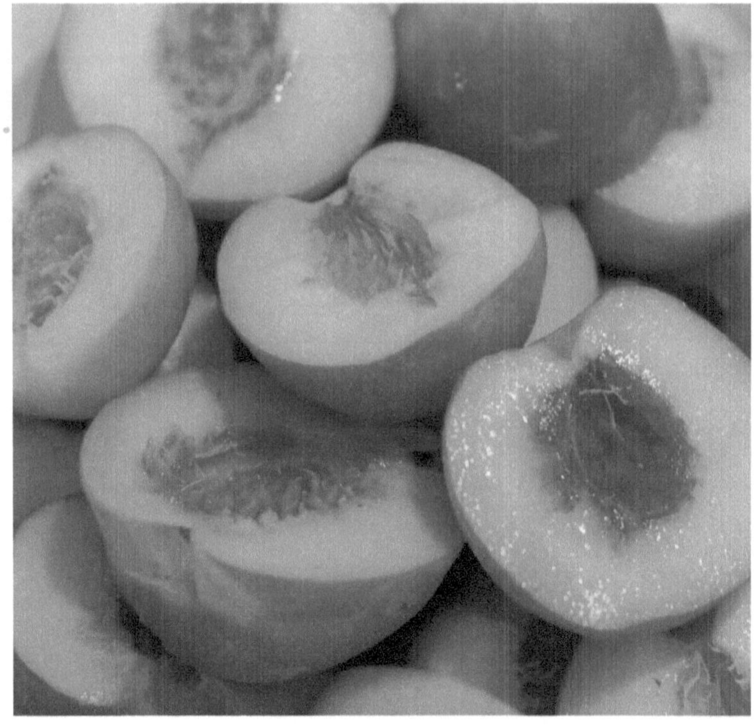

A nutritious and healthy recipe that combines fresh mint with nectarine.

Serves: 2

Time: 7 mins.

Ingredients:

- Nectarine (1, pitted, fresh)
- Carrots (8, fresh, washed)
- lettuce (2 handfuls, red, torn)
- Lime (½, fresh, peeled)
- Mint (2 sprigs, fresh)

Directions:

1. Thoroughly wash ingredients under water and use hands to scrub.

2. In a juicer add freshly washed ingredients and begin to juice.

3. Pour mixture into a tall glass, chill and serve immediately.

Sweet Potato Juice

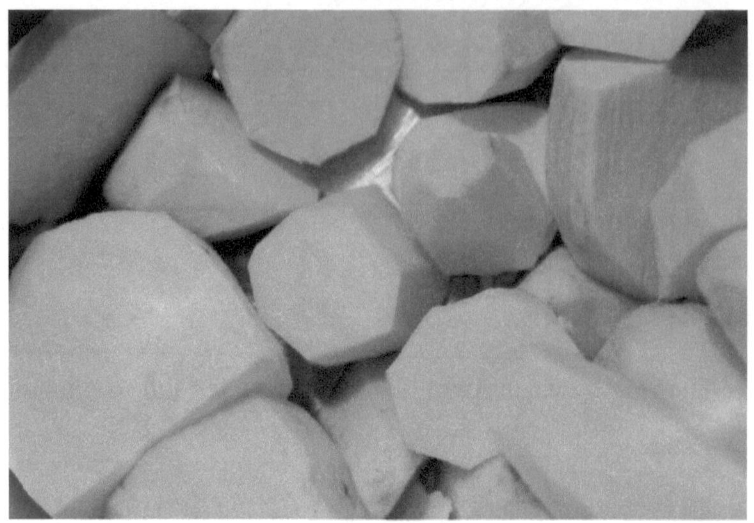

A tasty naturally sweetened potato juice recipe loaded with antioxidants.

Serves: 1

Time: 3 mins.

Ingredients:

- Potato (1, sweet, large, peeled)
- Apples (2, red, cored)
- Orange (1, fresh, peeled)
- Carrot (1, large, peeled)
- Celery (4 stalks, Fresh)
- Turmeric (1 piece, large, peeled)

Directions:

1. Thoroughly wash ingredients under water and use hands to scrub.

2. In a juicer add freshly washed ingredients and begin to juice.

3. Pour mixture into a tall glass, chill and serve immediately.

Best Weight Loss Juice

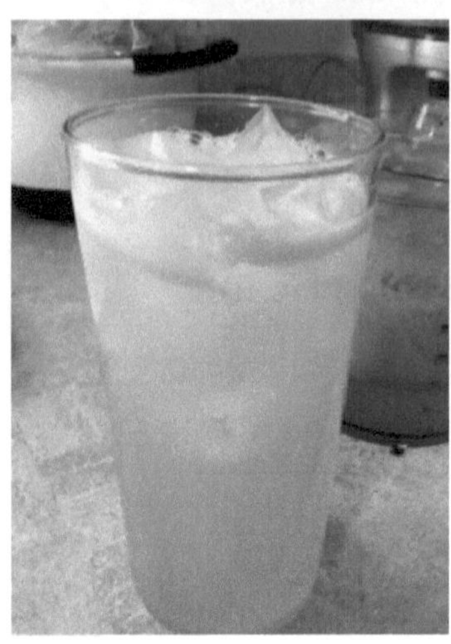

A healthy concoction which combines turmeric with pineapple and fresh vegetables. A combination guaranteed for weight loss.

Serves: 2

Time: 7 mins.

Ingredients:

- Pineapple (¼, fresh, peeled)
- Kale (4 leaves, Large)
- Celery (2 stalks)
- Lettuce (4 leaves, large)
- Parsley (1 bunch Flat, fresh)
- Lemon (1 lemon, fresh, peeled)
- Ginger (1 piece, fresh, peeled)
- Turmeric (1 piece, fresh, peeled)
- Chilies (1-2, for taste)

Directions:

1. Thoroughly wash ingredients under water and use hands to scrub.

2. In a juicer add freshly washed ingredients and begin to juice.

3. Pour mixture into a tall glass, chill and serve immediately.

Celery Eggplant

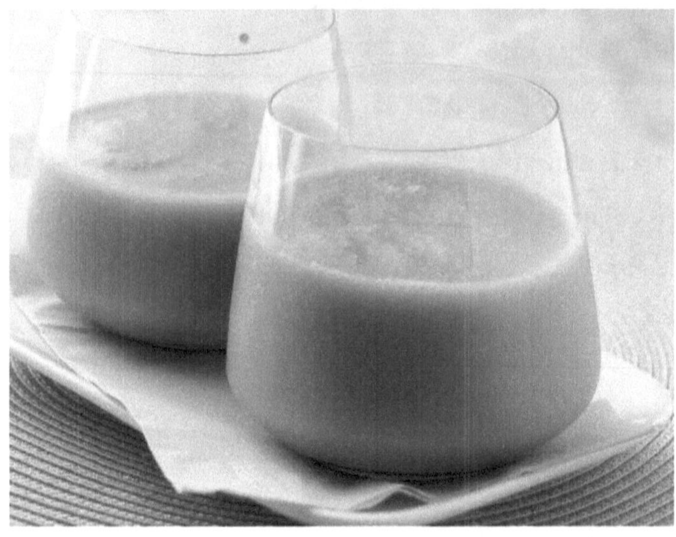

Celery Eggplant juice is widely known for its cholesterol curing properties, it also has great detox properties.

Serves: 2

Time: 10 mins.

Ingredients:

- Apricot (1)
- Celery (2 ribs)
- Eggplant (1)
- Pineapple (½)
- Wheatgrass (½ handful)
- Garlic (1 clove)
- Asparagus (2 spears)
- Beet (½)
- Papaya (½)

Directions:

1. Thoroughly wash ingredients under water and use hands to scrub.

2. In a juicer, add freshly washed ingredients and begin to juice.

3. Pour mixture into a tall glass, chill and serve immediately.

Conclusion

You did it! Congratulations on cooking your way to the end of this International Detox Juice Cookbook. Hopefully, you found all 30 of these tasty Detox Juice recipes easy to follow and tasty!

Now, with these 30 Detox Juice recipes added to your arsenal of drinks, you should be able to mix and match the ingredients to create even other delicious creations that are all tasty and intriguing.

Ensure to leave us a review if you liked what you read. Join us again for yet another delicious journey.

About the Author

Born in New Germantown, Pennsylvania, Stephanie Sharp received a Masters degree from Penn State in English Literature. Driven by her passion to create culinary masterpieces, she applied and was accepted to The International Culinary School of the Art Institute where she excelled in French cuisine. She has married her cooking skills with an aptitude for business by opening her own small cooking school where she teaches students of all ages.

Stephanie's talents extend to being an author as well and she has written over 400 e-books on the art of cooking and baking that include her most popular recipes.

Sharp has been fortunate enough to raise a family near her hometown in Pennsylvania where she, her husband and children live in a beautiful rustic house on an extensive piece of land. Her other passion is taking care of the furry members of her family which include 3 cats, 2 dogs and a potbelly pig named Wilbur.

Watch for more amazing books by Stephanie Sharp coming out in the next few months.

Author's Afterthoughts

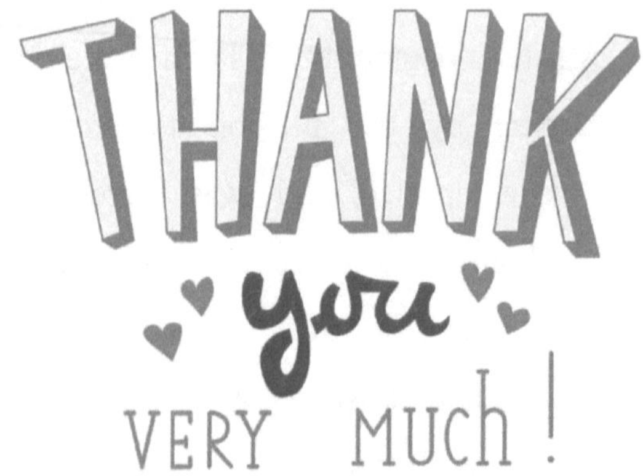

I am truly grateful to you for taking the time to read my book. I cherish all of my readers! Thanks ever so much to each of my cherished readers for investing the time to read this book!

With so many options available to you, your choice to buy my book is an honour, so my heartfelt thanks at reading it from beginning to end!

I value your feedback, so please take a moment to submit an honest and open review on Amazon so I can get valuable insight into my readers' opinions and others can benefit from your experience.

Thank you for taking the time to review!

Stephanie Sharp